Published By Robert Corbin

@ George Harris

Go Vegan: Everything You Need to an Awesome

Lifestyle - With Delicious Recipes and Lose

Weight, Diet, Diabetes, Fitness, Heart Disease,

Good Health

All Right RESERVED

ISBN 978-1-7385954-6-4

TABLE OF CONTENTS

Banana Bread 1

Black Beans... 3

Vegan Green Olive Tapenade... 6

Vegan Stuffed Mushroom 8

Berry Almond Breakfast Quinoa..................................... 10

Carrot Cake Quinoa Bars 12

Carrot Dog 16

Lentil Roast With Balsamic Onion Gravy........................ 18

Vegan Sausage Rolls 21

Detox Salad 24

Loaded Veggie Tofu Pie 27

Oatmeal Bowl.. 29

Vegan Chocolate Rice Crispiest 31

Raw Cookie Dough Balls 33

Pasta With Mushrooms.. 35

Chickpea Curry 38

Vegan Herb Spreadale Dip 41

- Vegan Rice Paper Rolls 43
- Oven-Baked Beans 45
- Strawberry Banana Spinach Smoothie 48
- Onion Rings 50
- No-Beef And Broccoli 51
- Vegan Spinach Ricotta Lasagna 53
- Easy Banana-Cacao Ice Cream 56
- Protein Blueberry Bars 58
- Vegan Philly Cheeses Teak 60
- Steamed Eggplant And Mushrooms With Peanut Sauce 62
- Baked Oatmeal 64
- French Toast Surprise 66
- Special Banana Pancakes 68
- Cauliflower Curry 70
- Corn Enchiladas 72
- Vegan Pull Apart Bread 76
- Vegan Jalapeno Poppers 78
- Scrambled Tofu Tacos 80

- Tofu Quiche 83
- Chickpea Nuggets 87
- Bean Tacos 89
- Chickpea Scramble Breakfast Basin 91
- Vegan Smoothie 93
- Quinoa, Oats, Hazelnut And Blueberry Salad 95
- Tofu Club Sandwich 98
- Italian–Style Spaghetti Squash With Tempe 100
- Mexican Zucchini Casserole 102
- Healthy Baked Eggplant Fries 105
- Simple Tofu Scramble 108
- Lentil Soup 110
- Carrot Soup With Pistachios 113
- Vegan Tteokbokki 116
- Vegan Creamy Cucumber 118
- Banana Quinoa Bars 120
- Overnight Oats With Fruits 123
- Sheet Pan Veggies 125

Vegan Chilli 127

Kiwi Fruit Smoothie 129

Protein Breakfast Burrito 130

Vegan Cheesy Sc2s 134

Dilled Chickpea Burger With Spicy Yogurt Sauce 137

Lovely Vegan Flapjacks 140

Mac & Cheese 142

Quinoa Soup 145

Pumpkin Soup 148

Vegan Spanakopita 150

Vegan Loaded Potato Bites 152

Banana Bread

Ingredients:

- ½ Cup of applesauce
- 1 Teaspoon of baking soda
- 1 Teaspoon of salt
- 1 Teaspoon of cinnamon
- 1 tablespoon of chopped walnuts
- 2 Medium ripe bananas
- 1 Peeled and diced apple
- ½ Cup of sugar
- 1 and ¾ cups of whole-wheat flour

Directions:

1. Preheat your oven to about 350°F. Grease a medium loaf pan with vegetable oil
2. In a medium bowl, mash your bananas with a fork.
3. Add the sugar, the diced apple, the flour, the applesauce, the baking soda, the salt, and the cinnamon to your bowl, and mix it very well.
4. Pour your Ingredients: to your prepared greased pan; then sprinkle with the chopped walnuts
5. Bake for about 50 minutes
6. Remove the bread from the oven and set it aside for around 15 minutes
7. Serve and enjoy your bread!

Black Beans

Ingredients:

- ½ teaspoon of salt

- 4 pressed garlic cloves

- 2 tablespoons of chili powder

- 2 teaspoons of ground cumin

- 1 and ½ teaspoons of smoked paprika

- 1 teaspoon of dried oregano

- 1 large can of diced tomatoes

- 2 cans of rinsed black beans

- 1 can of pinto rinsed beans

- 2 cups of water

- 2 bay leaves

- 2 tablespoons of chopped fresh cilantro
- 2 teaspoons of lime juice
- 1 peeled and sliced avocado
- Tortilla chips
- 2 tablespoons of olive oil
- 1 medium chopped red onion
- 1 large chopped red bell pepper
- 2 chopped medium carrots
- 2 chopped ribs of celery
- Grated cheese and sour cream

Directions:

1. In a heavy pot and over a medium heat, heat the olive oil until it shimmers.

2. Add your chopped onion, the bell pepper, the carrot, the celery and ¼ teaspoon of salt.
3. Stir very well to from time to time and cook for 10 minutes
4. Add the chili powder, the garlic, the cumin, the smoked paprika and the oregano.
5. Cook your Ingredients: until it becomes fragrant and keep stirring for 2 minutes
6. Add your diced tomatoes with its juices; add the rinsed and drained black beans and the pinto beans
7. Add the water and the bay leaf; then stir very well to combine it. Cook the mixture for about 30 minutes.
8. Remove your chili from the heat and transfer and add the cilantro and the vinegar
9. Add the salt; serve your chili with garnishes of your choice
10. Enjoy your chili!

Vegan Green Olive Tapenade

Ingredients:

- 2 tbsp. capers
- 2 tbsp. dried tomatoes
- ½ cup chopped parsley
- 1 tsp. Bragg's liquid amino
- 2 tbsp. olive oil
- ¾ cup green olives
- ½ cup almond (soaked)
- 1 garlic clove
- Vegan crackers

Directions:

1. Add all the Ingredients: in a food processor except crackers and process it until forms well combined paste.
2. Serve it with vegan crackers!

Vegan Stuffed Mushroom

Ingredients:

- 1-2 garlic clove grated
- Crushed red pepper to taste
- Salt to taste
- 1 tbsp. olive oil
- ½ tbsp. chopped parsley
- 5-6 whole mushroom (washed and remove stems)
- 2-3 mushroom chopped
- ¼ cup panko bread crumbs

Directions:

1. Preheat oven to 400° F

2. Heat oil in a pan; add garlic, chopped mushroom, red pepper and salt, cook it for 2-3 sec.
3. Then add crumbs and mix it well.
4. Turn off the flame and allow it to cool.
5. Fill mushrooms with the prepared stuffing and place it on lined baking sheet.
6. Bake it for 20 min and garnish with chopped parsley.

Berry Almond Breakfast Quinoa

Ingredients:

- 5 cups of mixed berries
- A quarter tsp. of cardamom (ground)
- 3 cups of milk (almond)
- 5 tbsps. almonds (sliced)
- 3 tbsps. maple syrup
- Half a tsp. cinnamon (ground)
- 2 cup of quinoa

Directions:

1. Take a medium-sized pot and add quinoa, cinnamon, almond milk, and cardamom to it. Mix the Ingredients: well.

2. Apply the heat to the pot so that the contents start to boil.
3. After the boiling has started turn the regulator to low flame and let it stand for about fifteen minutes.
4. This will help the quinoa cook thoroughly.
5. Cool the quinoa and stir maple syrup into it.
6. Divide the cooked quinoa-maple syrup mixture into 5 containers. Each container should contain a three-5th cup of quinoa (cooked), 2 tbsp. of almonds (sliced) and 2 cup of fruit.
7. Instant pot- when you are using it, replace the almond milk with water.
8. Cook for about 2 minute on steep pressure. Allow it to release steam naturally.
9. Also, when using a rice cooker, put water into the cooker instead of almond milk.

Carrot Cake Quinoa Bars

Ingredients:

A quarter cup each of

- Hemp hearts

- Walnuts, chopped (keep some pieces aside for topping)

Half a cup each of

- A large-sized banana (mashed)

- Coconut sugar

- Carrots (grated)

- Apple sauce (unsweetened)

- Salt to taste

- Coconut butter-cream for frosting

Half a tsp. Each of

- Vanilla bean (ground), vanilla extract is also preferable

- Nutmeg (ground)

- Baking soda

- A three-5th cup of quinoa flour

- 2 cup of chickpeas (cooked)

- 2 tsp. of cinnamon (ground)

- 2 and a half tablespoons of flaxseed meal plus three tablespoons of water (2 flax egg)

Directions:

1. Keep the oven ready by setting its temperature at 350 degrees Fahrenheit/180 degrees Celsius. Use a baking pan and line its sides using parchment paper. Place the

parchment-lined baking pan on the oven and grease it with oil. The baking pan must be 8x8 in dimension.

2. Take a small bowl and add the flaxseed meal (the quantity that is menti2d in the Ingredients: section) and water to it. Whisk them properly to combine and set the mixture aside for about five minutes.

3. Use the five minutes to blend banana, applesauce, and chickpeas (cooked) in the bowl of a food processor until the mixture becomes fully smooth in texture.

4. Add all the raw Ingredients: (except carrot, hemp hearts, and walnut) to a large-sized mixing bowl and whisk them together using a fork. Assemble the mixture with the flaxseed meal and chickpea puree that you have just prepared. Fuse them well until all the Ingredients: incorporate.

5. Now gather the remaining Ingredients: that were reserved till now that is, hemp hearts, carrots (grated), and walnut slices into the bowl and blend well to combine.
6. After the batter is prepared, drain it into the pan (baking), which has already been set to bake. Place the pan on center rack and allow the batter to bake for about twenty-six minutes. This period should be enough to let a toothpick forced into the center to come out clean.
7. Allow it to cool for another fifteen minutes and then let it cool completely in a rack made of wire.
8. Cut it into sixteen bars and frost it with coconut butter-cream.

Carrot Dog

Ingredients:

Carrots & marinade

- Shave and BOIL carrots until tender (fork should easily go through then)

Marinade:

- 3 chopped shallots

- 3 tbsp liquid smoke

- 3 cloves chopped garlic

- ½ cup apple cider vinegar

- 3 tbsp garlic powder

- 3 tbsp onion powder

- 2 tbsp seas2d salt

- 1 tbsp salt/black pepper

- 1 cup water

Directions:

1. Leave carrots in marinade at least an hour PREFERABLY overnight
2. Remove from marinade and fry carrots over medium high heat rotating until outer edges are brown and slightly crisp. Grilling is also an option! Add to bun and accessorize

Lentil Roast With Balsamic Onion Gravy

Ingredients:

- 2 tbsps mixed dry herbs

- 1 cup red wine

- 14 oz cooked kidney beans, rinsed

- 3 tbsps balsamic vinegar

- 1 tbsp arrowroot powder

- 1 1/3 cup rolled oats

- 1 vegetable stock cube

- 4 tbsps yeast

- 1 red onion, sliced

- 3 tbsp vegetable oil

- 1 tbsp coconut sugar

- 3 garlic cloves, minced

- 2 portobello mushrooms, chopped

- 4 tbsps tamari soy sauce

- 1 onion, minced

- 14 oz cooked puy lentils, rinsed

- 1 carrot, grated

- Black pepper, to taste

Directions:

1. Preheat oven to 350f and prepare a can of lined bread.
2. Heat 1 tbsp of vegetable oil in a pan and cook the onion and garlic until soft.
3. Add the carrot and mushrooms and cook for 5 more minutes.

4. Add beans, puy lentils, 1 tbsp of tamari sauce, herbs, yeast, oatmeal and a little pepper and mash to combine. Transfer to bread pan and bake for 45 minutes.
5. Add 1/2 litre of vegetable stock with a bucket of stock and reserve. Add 2 tbsps of vegetable oil to a pan and add onion and coconut sugar and cook for 10 minutes.
6. Add arrowroot powder and stir to combine.
7. Add balsamic vinegar, wine and tamari sauce and cook until the broth is reduced.
8. Add the vegetable stock cube and cook for 10 minutes.
9. Serve with the loaf of bread.

Vegan Sausage Rolls

Ingredients:

- 70g fresh white breadcrumbs

- 2 tsp dijon mustard

- 250g chestnut mushrooms

- 1 tbsp brown rice miso

- 3 tsp olive oil

- 2 leeks, finely chopped

- 1 tbsp finely chopped rosemary leaves

- 1 x 320g sheet ready-rolled puff pastry

- 30g chestnuts, very finely chopped

- 2 big garlic cloves, crushed

- Dairy-free milk, to glaze

- Plain flour for dusting

Directions:

1. Add the mushrooms in a food processor and press until finely chopped.
2. Place half of the olive oil in a pan, add the leeks along with a pinch of salt and simmer for 15 minutes or until soft and golden brown.
3. Scrape the leeks into a bowl and allow to cool slightly.
4. Heat the rest of the oil in the pan and then fry the mushrooms for 10 minutes over medium heat.
5. Add garlic, sage, miso and mustard, and simmer for another minute. Cool slightly.
6. Heat the toaster in a 200c.
7. Add the mushroom mixture in the bowl with the leeks, then add the chestnuts and breadcrumbs.

8. Season, then combine everything together until you get a slightly stiff mixture.
9. Untangle the pastry on a floured surface, then spread the pastry outwards to ensure that a single side sways 43 cm.
10. Mould the sausage-shaped mushroom and leek mixture in the centre of the dough, then place the dough around the filling and then turn along the seam with a fork.
11. Cut into ten pieces. Place a baking sheet lined with parchment and brush each piece with milk.
12. Bake for 25 minutes or until golden brown and deep.
13. Let cool slightly and sprinkle with sesame seeds before serving.

Detox Salad

Ingredients:

- 1 bunch kale, de-stemmed and chopped into bite size pieces

- 1 small head red cabbage, chopped into bite size pieces

- 1 cup cooked black beans

- 2 large or 4 small roasted beets, chopped into bite size pieces

- 2 cups roasted Brussels sprouts

- 1 avocado, peeled, pitted, sliced

- 8 ounces spring mix

- 4 carrots, chopped

- 4 Portobello caps, chopped
- 1 cup red bell pepper, chopped
- ½ cup raw sunflower seeds For balsamic

Dressing:

- 2 teaspoons Dijon mustard
- Juice of a lemon
- 4 tablespoons olive oil
- 1 teaspoon minced garlic
- Sea salt to taste
- ½ cup balsamic vinegar
- 4 tablespoons maple syrup
- Pepper to taste

Directions:

1. To make the dressing: Add all the Ingredients: of the dressing in a bowl. Whisk well.
2. Add mushrooms into it and toss well. Let it marinate in it overnight or at least for 3-4 hours.
3. Transfer to a large serving bowl. Add kale, spring mix, cabbage, carrots, black beans, beets and red pepper. Toss well. Refrigerate until use.
4. To serve: divide and serve the salad in individual serving bowls.
5. Add Brussels sprouts, avocado and sunflower seeds on top and serve.

Loaded Veggie Tofu Pie

Ingredients:

- 8 spring onions, chopped

- ¼ cup nutritional yeast

- 2 cups carrots, chopped

- 2 cups celery leaves, chopped 2 medium tomatoes, sliced Black pepper powder to taste

- ¼ cup olive oil

- ¼ cup low sodium soy sauce

- 2 blocks extra firm tofu, crumbled

- 5 tablespoons Dijon mustard or to taste

- 4 cups fresh spinach, chopped

- 1 cup yellow or orange bell pepper, chopped
- 1 cup red bell pepper, chopped

Directions:

1. Spray a baking dish with cooking spray.
2. Add mustard, bell peppers, soy sauce, spinach, carrots, onions, tofu, and celery into the baking dish.
3. Mix well and press well on to the bottom of the dish.
4. Place tomato slices on top and sprinkle nutritional yeast.
5. Bake in a preheated oven at 400°F for 45-60 minutes.
6. Slice into wedges and serve.

Oatmeal Bowl

Ingredients:

- 1 tablespoon peanut or almond butter

- 1 tablespoon shelled hemp seeds or chia seeds

- ½ teaspoon ground cinnamon

- ¼ teaspoon sea salt

- ½ cup rolled oats

- 1 cup boiling water

- 2 tablespoons raisins or unsweetened dried cranberries (optional)

- Splash of maple syrup

Directions:

1. Boil water, add oats, and reduce to a simmer.
2. Stir in raisins or cranberries, if using.
3. Continue to simmer for 10-15 minutes or until oats are tender and raisins or cranberries are plumped.
4. While the oatmeal is still in the hot pan, stir in peanut or almond butter, hemp or chia seeds, cinnamon, and sea salt. Serve lightly drizzled with maple syrup.

Vegan Chocolate Rice Crispiest

Ingredients:

- 4 tbsp. hemp seeds

- 4 cups puffed rice cereal

- 4 cups puffed kamut cereal

- 10 oz vegan marshmallow creme

- 1/4 cup cocoa

- 2 tbsp. chia seeds

- 6 tbsp. fresh-brewed coffee or water

- 1/2 cup vegan chocolate chips

Directions:

1. Combine the chia seeds and coffee or water in a small bowl, stir and set aside until thickened.
2. In a large bowl, combine the hemp seeds, puffed rice and puffed kamut cereals. Set aside.
3. Prepare a pan and line it with parchment paper.
4. In a large saucepan, gently warm the marshmallow creme, cocoa and chocolate chips, stirring to thoroughly melt the chocolate chips.
5. When the mixture is melted and combined, pour it into the cereal mixture and stir until all of the cereal is coated with the chocolate mixture.
6. Pour the cereal/chocolate mixture into the pan and place in the refrigerator until set.
7. Cut into squares and Serve.

Raw Cookie Dough Balls

Ingredients:

- 3 tbsp maple syrup (or agave syrup)
- 2 tbsp coconut oil
- 1 tsp vanilla extract
- ½ cup vegan chocolate chips
- 1 cup oats (use gluten-free oats as required)
- 1 ripe banana
- ½ cup grated dry unsweetened coconut

Directions:

1. In a food processor, add the oats, and pulse for 20 seconds in order to break the oats down slightly.
2. Add the rest of the Ingredients: (EXCEPT the chocolate chips) and pulse until fully combined.
3. Stir-in the chocolate chips.
4. Roll into 12 balls and refrigerate for 1 hour.
5. Store in an airtight container in the fridge.

Pasta With Mushrooms

Ingredients:

- 3 minced and divided garlic cloves

- 1 and ½ cups of vegan marinara sauce

- 2 cup of water

- 2 and ¼ teaspoon of sea salt more

- 1 teaspoon of ground black pepper

- 12 oz of dry pasta

- ½ of small cubed eggplant

- 2 cups of cremini or button sliced mushrooms

- 2 tablespoon of olive oil

Directions:

1. Rinse your eggplant and dice it into small cubes
2. Put the eggplant in your sink and sprinkle it with salt; then set it aside for 30 minutes
3. Rinse the eggplant and dry it with a clean towel.
4. Put a saucepan over a medium heat and add 3 tbsp of olive oil to your eggplant with 1 minced garlic clove.
5. Add ½ teaspoon of sea salt and stir very well; then sauté your Ingredients: for about 5 minutes or until it becomes golden brown. Stir in the mushrooms and cook it for 2 more minutes. Set the Ingredients: aside.
6. In your saucepan, add the water, the pasta, the marinara sauce and the remaining garlic cloves.
7. Add 1 and ½ teaspoons of sea salt with 1 teaspoon of black pepper

8. Boil the mixture and set it aside to simmer for about 10 minutes.
9. Adjust your seasoning and add salt and herbs
10. Remove the pasta from the heat and top it with the mixture of the eggplant and the mushroom; then add the parsley or the basil
11. Serve and enjoy!

Chickpea Curry

Ingredients:

- 3 Garlic cloves

- ½ a lime

- 2 Tbsp of Masala curry paste

- 1 and ½ cups of coconut milk

- 1 Can of drained and rinsed chickpeas

- 2 Tablespoons of soy sauce

- 3 Medium chopped cherry tomatoes

- 1 Cup of basil leaves

- ½ Cup of basmati rice

- 1 Cup of water

- 2 Pinches of salt

- 2 Medium diced onions

- 2 Tbsp of olive oil

- 1 Teaspoon of maple syrup

Directions:

1. In a saucepan, pour the water, the rice, 1 pinch of salt and bring the Ingredients: to a boil
2. Reduce the heat and cook for about 10 minutes; stir from time to time; meanwhile, cut the onions into dices, cut the garlic, the basil and the lime.
3. Place the oil and add the onions to a pan and cook it on a medium heat for around 5 minutes
4. Add the garlic cloves and cook for 1 minute

5. Add 1 tablespoon of curry paste and pour the milk; make sure to stir from time to time Add 1 pinch of salt; then add the chickpeas
6. Pour in the soy sauce, and cook all of your Ingredients: for about 5 minutes and when it starts boiling, reduce the heat
7. Add the tomatoes, the chopped basil and the lime juice; then let simmer the curry for about 2 minutes.
8. Taste your curry again and add 1 tbsp of soy sauce; then pour in the brown sugar and stir
9. Serve and enjoy your curry with naan bread

Vegan Herb Spreadale Dip

Ingredients:

- 1 cup cashew nuts (soaked)

- 2 tbsp. lemon juice

- 1 tbsp. nutritional yeast

- 3-4 garlic cloves (roasted)

- Salt to taste

- Pomegranate seeds for garnishing

- 4 tbsp. mix herb chopped (desired combination)

- 3 tbsp. full fat coconut milk

- Vegan crackers for serving

Directions:

1. Add all the Ingredients: in a food processor and process it until forms well combined paste.
2. Wrap it in cheesecloth and place it in a desired shape bowl.
3. Cover with plastic wrap and keep in fridge for overnight.
4. Garnish with pomegranate seeds and serve with crackers.

Vegan Rice Paper Rolls

Ingredients:

- Italian seasoning to taste

- Salt to taste

- Water as needed

- 1 cup mix veggies (desired)

- ¼ cup beans (desired and cooked)

- 5-6 rice paper

Directions:

1. Cut veggies into thin strips.
2. Heat a pan; add veggies, seasoning and salt in it.
3. Stir fry veggies using splash of water.
4. Now add beans and mix it well.
5. Turn off the flame and allow it to cool.

6. Wet the rice paper and dry it.
7. Place vegetables on it and wrap it.
8. Enjoy!

Oven-Baked Beans

Ingredients:

- 3 tablespoons of balsamic vinegar

- 2 jar of tomato passata (about 700 milliliters)

- 2 tablespoon of olive oil

- Three cloves of garlic, peeled

- Three to five sprigs of thyme (fresh)

- 3 tins of pinto beans (about 5teen ounces or 397 grams)

- Half a teaspoon of cumin (ground)

- 2 de-seeded red chili

- 2 teaspoon each of

- Molasses

- Paprika (smoked)

- Chili flakes

- 3 onions (red)

Directions:

1. Heat the oven beforehand by setting its temperature to 170 degrees Celsius/338 degrees Fahrenheit.
2. Make thin slices of the onion. Make fine slices of the garlic and chili.
3. You will require a roasting tray which is oven proof and large-sized.
4. Place all the chopped Ingredients: into the roasting tray, add spices as instructed in the Ingredients: section and dress with olive oil.
5. Mix them up using a spoon and cover the tray with foil paper.

6. Place the tray over the oven and let the mixture roast for about twenty minutes.
7. After this span, add the remaining Ingredients: to the tray and sauté carefully.
8. Before adding the second round of Ingredients:, make sure to remove the tray from the oven.
9. Put it back to the oven and roast for another forty-five minutes, without covering.
10. Take the tray out of the oven and sauté. To make the sauce less condensed, add about a quarter cup of water.

Strawberry Banana Spinach Smoothie

Ingredients:

- 5 teaspoons of chia seeds

- Half cup of almond milk (unsweetened)

- 3 tablespoons of protein powder (vanilla flavored)

- 5 cups of fresh spinach

- 3 cups each of

- Sliced bananas (frozen)

- Whole strawberries (frozen)

Directions:

1. Line a baking sheet with parchment paper.
2. Spread all the sliced bananas and whole strawberries on the baking sheet and then

keep it in the freezer for 3 hours until it gets frozen completely.
3. Write the date and Strawberry Banana Spinach Smoothie on the front of 5 quart-sized freezer bags.
4. Add a handful of spinach, a cup of frozen fruits, and 2 teaspoon of chia seeds into each freezer bag.
5. Squeeze all the air out of the bags before sealing them in order to prevent freezer burn.
6. Seal the bags and keep them in the freezer for use later on.
7. When you want to have the smoothie, pour the entire content of the strawberry banana spinach smoothie bag into a high-speed blender.
8. Add half cup of almond milk and 3 tablespoons of protein powder into the blender and blend everything on high for about a minute so that everything is blended.

Onion Rings

Ingredients:

- 1 large yellow onion
- 1 ½ cup plant milk
- 1 cup chickpea flour
- Frying oil
- Seasonings: salt/pepper/ garlic powder/ cayenne

Directions:

1. Mix flour, plant milk and seasonings into batter.
2. Place each ring into batter then deep fry for about 1-2 minutes per side.

No-Beef And Broccoli

Ingredients:

- 1 head of broccoli (chopped)

- 1 cup baby Portobello mushrooms ½ cup chopped onion Seasonings:

- Salt / pepper to taste

- ½ cup Soy sauce 1 tbsp cornstarch 3 tbsp water

Directions:

1. In a non stick pan add mushrooms with a pinch of salt.
2. Sauté for a minute or 2. Next add broccoli with about 2 tbsp of water and cover to steam about 5 minutes, stirring occasionally.
3. Mix cornstarch and 3 tbsp water in a separate container.

4. Pour soy sauce and cornstarch mixture into the pan with mushroom and broccoli.
5. Stir, season to taste with salt and pepper.
6. Allow to simmer for about 3 minutes.

Vegan Spinach Ricotta Lasagna

Ingredients:

- 2 lemons, juiced

- 1 tsp salt

- 1/3 cup flour

- 2 tsp dried oregano

- 3/4 cup passata

- 2 tbsps olive oil

- A pinch black pepper

- 3 cup soy sauce

- 1 lb frozen spinach

- 1 tbsp mustard

- 2/3 lb lasagna sheets

- 1/3 cup margarine

- 1 lb firm tofu

- 5 garlic cloves

- A pinch nutmeg

Directions:

1. Defrost the spinach. Add olive oil, garlic cloves, lemon juice, nutmeg, mustard, black pepper and 1/2 tsp of salt to a blender and mix until smooth.
2. Break the tofu into pieces and add them to the blender. Blend until it's smooth.
3. Melt the margarine in a pan, add the flour and mix well. Add soy milk and 1/2 tsp of salt and continue beating.
4. Mix the passata, dried oregano, salt and pepper in a bowl.

5. Prepare the lasagna starting with a layer of lasagna noodles and cover with the tofu mixture. Pour over with the sauce.
6. Cover the last lasagna sheet with both sauces to completely cover the pasta — bake for 40 minutes at 375 f.
7. Serve and enjoy.

Easy Banana-Cacao Ice Cream

Ingredients:

- 1 tsp maple syrup
- 1 scoop vegan chocolate pr otein powder
- 1 tsp maca powder
- 1 tbsp raw cacao powder
- 2 tsps natural peanut butter
- 2 bananas, frozen
- Almonds, chopped
- Cacao nibs
- Chia seeds
- Pinch cinnamon

- Ground flax seeds

- Splash almond milk

Directions:

1. Blend all Ingredients: except cacao nibs, ground flax seeds, chia seeds, and almonds in a blender on high speed.
2. Transfer the mixture to a container and place it into the freezer. Freeze for about 4-8 hours, stirring every 1 hour.
3. Serve topped with ground flax seeds, chia seeds, cacao nibs, and almonds.

Protein Blueberry Bars

Ingredients:

- 1 ½ cups rolled oats
- 1/3 cup ground flaxseed
- ½ cup pistachios
- ¼ cup apple sauce
- 1 cup almond butter
- 1/3 cup pipits
- 1/3 cup walnuts
- ¾ cup whole almonds
- ½ cup dried blueberries
- 1/3 cup maple syrup

Directions:

1. In a bowl, mix rolled oats, blueberries, almonds, flaxseed, nuts, sunflower seeds, pistachios and nuggets.
2. Add apple sauce and maple syrup.
3. Mix the almond butter, then pour the dough into a baking sheet lined with parchment paper (the paper should be large enough to cover and rim over the edges of the baking sheet).
4. Press the dough firmly with the palms of your hands and then spread it evenly.
5. Refrigerate for 1 hour. Remove from the freezer then and lift the dough from the mould by lifting the paper.
6. Place on a work surface and gently remove the paper. Cut the dough into 16 bars and serve.

Vegan Philly Cheeses Teak

Ingredients:

- ½ teaspoon garlic powder

- ½ teaspoon onion powder 2 blocks (7 ounces each) dairy free Provol2 style cheese slices 2 green pepper, deseeded, sliced

- 2 packages (8 ounce each) seaman (vegan meat)

- 2 teaspoons celery flakes

- ½ cup olive oil

- 1 medium yellow onions, sliced

- Salt to taste

- Pepper to taste

- 4 vegan French rolls, halved lengthwise

Directions:

1. Place a large pan over medium heat. Add 4 tablespoons olive oil.
2. When the oil is heated, add green pepper, seaman and onion and sauté until the seaman is thoroughly heated.
3. Add onion powder, garlic powder, celery flakes, salt and pepper and mix well.
4. Turn off the heat and add into a baking dish.
5. Place cheese slices on top.
6. 5. Bake in a preheated oven at 375°F for 10 to 15 minutes or until the cheese melts.
7. Place another pan over medium heat. Add remaining oil.
8. Cook the French rolls with the cut side facing down until brown and crisp.
9. Top rolls with the baked seaman filling and serve.

Steamed Eggplant And Mushrooms With Peanut Sauce

Ingredients:

- 1 tablespoon light brown sugar

- Coarse salt to taste

- Cooked rice, to serve (optional)

- ½ pound shiitake mushrooms, stems discarded, caps halved 1 ½ tablespoons rice vinegar

- 1 tablespoon, peeled, fresh ginger, finely grated

- 3 Japanese eggplants sliced into 1-inch-thick rounds

- 1 ½ tablespoons smooth peanut butter

- 1 tablespoon soy sauce

- 2 scallions, cut into 2-inch lengths, thinly sliced lengthwise

Directions:

1. Place a pot over medium heat. Pour enough water to cover an inch from the bottom of the pot.
2. Add eggplant and mushrooms. Steam the eggplant and mushrooms for a few minutes until tender. Transfer to a bowl.
3. Add peanut butter and vinegar into a small bowl and whisk until smooth.
4. Add rest of the Ingredients: and whisk well.
5. Add this to the bowl of eggplants. Add scallions and toss.
6. Serve hot with rice.

Baked Oatmeal

Ingredients:

- 2 tsp. Baking powder
- 1 tsp. Cinnamon
- 1/2 cup raisins
- 6 tbsp. Unsweetened applesauce*
- 1/2 cup oil
- 1 cup "milk"
- 3 cups quick oats
- 1/2 cup sugar
- 1/2 tsp. Salt
- Margarine (for greasing baking dish)

Directions:

1. Preheat oven to 350 degrees. Lightly grease a 2-quart glass casserole dish with margarine.
2. In a bowl, stir together all dry Ingredients:.
3. Add wet Ingredients: and stir to combine.
4. Transfer to the casserole dish and cover. Bake for approx. 35 minutes.
5. Serve warm

French Toast Surprise

Ingredients:

- 1 1/2 teaspoon cinnamon
- 1 teaspoon pumpkin pie spice (optional)
- 1 teaspoon vanilla
- Bread, any kind is fine
- 2-3 ripe bananas
- 3/4 cup soy milk
- Vegan margarine

Directions:

1. Blend bananas, soy milk, cinnamon, pumpkin pie spice and vanilla in blender or food processor and pour mixture into pie plate or

wide dish. Gently dip bread slices into the mix, coating both sides.
2. Fry in vegan margarine in medium-hot skillet until golden brown.
3. Serve your French toast with maple syrup.

Special Banana Pancakes

Ingredients:

- 1 cup whole wheat flour
- 1/2 teaspoon salt
- 1 tablespoon ground flax
- 1 tablespoon applesauce
- 1/2 cup raspberries
- 2 bananas
- 1 tablespoon coconut oil
- 1 tablespoon brown rice syrup 1 teaspoon vanilla
- 1/2 cup water
- 3 teaspoons baking powder

Directions:

1. Mash bananas with a fork. Mix mashed bananas in a large mixing bowl with coconut oil, brown rice syrup, vanilla and water.
2. In a separate bowl, mix together baking powder, flour, salt and flax.
3. Combine dry Ingredients: with wet and whisk together.
4. Mix in applesauce, being sure not to kill all the poofiness the applesauce adds by over mixing.
5. Fold in the raspberries.
6. Scoop 1/4 up amounts of batter onto a hot, greased griddle.
7. Cook until golden brown on each side, about 5 minutes each.
8. Spatula onto a plate and serve immediately with maple syrup.

Cauliflower Curry

Ingredients:

- 1 Tablespoon of grated fresh ginger
- ¼ Cup of red curry paste
- 1 Can of coconut milk
- 1 Can of diced tomatoes
- 1 Head of cauliflower
- 1 and ½ teaspoons of Kosher salt
- 2 Tablespoons of vegetable oil
- 1 Small diced onion
- 1 Seeded and diced jalapeño
- 1 Pinch of fresh ground black pepper

Directions:

1. In a large saucepan, heat your oil over a medium heat.
2. Stir in the onion and the jalapeño; then cook the mixture until it becomes tender for 3 minutes
3. Stir in the ginger and cook your Ingredients:; stir from time to time
4. Add the curry paste and cook it for about 1 minute
5. Toss in the cauliflower florets with ½ cup of water.
6. Season your curry with 1 pinch of salt and 1 pinch of pepper.
7. Bring the Ingredients: to a boil and lower the heat and let it simmer until for 15 minutes
8. Serve and enjoy your cauliflower curry!

Corn Enchiladas

Ingredients:

- 4Oz of diced green

- 3 Small green onions

- ¼ Bunch of cilantro

- ¼ Teaspoon of salt

- 11 Corn tortillas

- 1 Medium zucchini

- 15 oz of drained black beans

- 1 Cup of frozen corn kernels

For the Enchilada Sauce

- 3Oz of tomato paste

- ½ Teaspoon of cumin

- ½ Teaspoon of garlic powder

- ¼ Teaspoon of cayenne pepper

- ¾ Teaspoon of salt

- 2 Tablespoons of vegetable oil

- 2 Tablespoons of chili powder

- 2 Tablespoons of flour

- 2 Cups of water

Directions:

1. Start by cutting the zucchini into tiny cubes; then rinse and drain your black beans.
2. Finely slice the green onions and chop the cilantro; then mix the zucchini with the black beans, the frozen corn kernels, the green onions, the cilantro, and the diced green chilies in a deep bowl.

3. Add around ¼ teaspoon of salt and then stir very well until it becomes evenly mixed.
4. To prepare the enchilada sauce, mix together the oil with the combine the chili powder and the flour into a medium sauce pan. Whisk your Ingredients: together over a medium heat and let it bubble
5. Pour in the water, the tomato paste, the cumin, the garlic, the cayenne and the salt
6. Whisk your Ingredients: until they become smooth and heat the enchilada sauce for about 4 minutes
7. Preheat your oven to about 350°F and grease a baking tray with oil
8. Pour ½ cup of your sauce into the tray, and line 1/3 the quantity of the tortillas
9. Pour in 1/3 of your vegetable mature and pour the rest of the vegetable sauce over the tortillas

10. Repeat the same process with until you finish the sauce; then bake the Ingredients: for about 40 minutes
11. Remove from the oven; top with onion slices; then serve and enjoy your enchiladas!

Vegan Pull Apart Bread

Ingredients:

- Vegan pizza dough (2 cups all-purpose flour+ 2 tbsp. olive oil+ 2 tsp. dry yeast+ 1 tsp. sugar+ 1 tsp. salt+ warm water as needed)

- Vegan pesto (2 cups basil+ 2-3 tbsp. walnuts+3 garlic cloves+ 2 tbsp. lemon juice+ 3 tbsp. nutritional yeast+ sea salt to taste+ 1tbsp. extra virgin olive oil+ water as needed- process in a food processor to make a smooth paste.)

- Flour for dusting

Directions:

1. Preheat oven to 400° F.

2. Take dough and roll it out in a large rectangle shape.
3. Spread pesto over it and cut into strips.
4. Layer each strip on top of other and then cut it into groups.
5. Place it into baking pan and bake it for 25- 30 minutes.

Vegan Jalapeno Poppers

Ingredients:

- 1 tsp. cumin powder
- salt and black pepper to taste
- 1 tbsp. cilantro chopped
- 7-8 jalapenos
- 1 tbsp. panko bread crumbs
- ¾ cup vegan cream cheese
- 1 garlic clove grated
- 1 tbsp. red onion chopped
- 1 chipotle chopped in adobo sauce

Directions:

1. Preheat oven to 400° F.

2. Mix all Ingredients: except jalapeno and crumbs.
3. Cut the jalapeno into 3 halves. (lengthwise)
4. Remove seeds and ribs, stuff it with prepared stuffing.
5. Now place it on baking sheet and sprinkle bread crumbs over it.
6. Bake it for 25- 30 minutes.

Scrambled Tofu Tacos

Ingredients:

- Eight corn tortillas (you can also use whole-grain tortillas)

- Half cup of grape tomatoes, quartered (you can also use diced Roma tomatoes)

- 2 clove of garlic, minced

- 2 avocado, sliced

- Black pepper, freshly ground

- 2-5th teaspoon each of

- Salt

- 2 pack of super firm Nasoya Tofu

- 2 red pepper, diced

- Ground turmeric

- Cumin

- Hot sauce and cilantro for garnish (optional)

- Half cup of goat cheese, crumbled (optional)

Directions:

1. Place a large skillet over medium heat and add some oil into it.
2. Add the diced red pepper and minced garlic into it and sauté for 3 minutes.
3. Crumble the tofu using your hands and add it to the skillet.
4. Add in the spices and season with salt and black pepper.
5. Cook it for about five minutes and stir frequently.
6. You can add more salt and pepper if you need.
7. Divide the scrambled tofu mixture equally between the tortillas.

8. Add the sliced avocados, tomatoes, and crumbled goat cheese as a topping and the hot sauce and cilantro as a garnish.

Tofu Quiche

Ingredients:

For the crust

- 3 tablespoons of melted vegan butter (Alternatively use olive oil)

- Three medium to large-sized potatoes (grated/You get three cups grated potatoes from three potatoes)

- A quarter teaspoon of pepper and sea salt

For the filling

- 3 medium leeks (Sliced thin, and cleaned completely, and dried/ Alternatively, for 3 leeks, 2 medium-sized onion can be diced and used)

- Three tablespoons of hummus

- Three-quarters cup of cherry tomatoes (Cut into halves)

- Black pepper, sea salt to suit your taste

- 3 tablespoons of nutritional yeast

- Three cloves of garlic (Chopped)

- 13 oz./352 g of extra-firm silken tofu (Pat dried)

- 2 cup of broccoli (Chopped)

Directions:

1. Switch on the oven to preheat it. The temperature should be 450 degrees Fahrenheit/230 degrees Celsius. Take a 9.5-inch pie pan, and spray non-stick cooking spray on it.
2. Grate the potatoes, and you need to use three cups of it. In a clean towel, place the grated

potatoes, and squeeze out the moisture, firmly. Transfer it to the pie pan. Over it dash the melted butter. Season with salt and pepper. The grated potatoes should get an even coat, so toss and press with your fingers. Compress against the sides and bottom of the pan.

3. Bake until the Ingredients: get golden brown fully. This can take around twenty-five to thirty minutes. Lower the heat to 400 degrees Fahrenheit/200 degrees Celcius, and take out the crust. Leave aside.

4. Prep the garlic and vegetables, and place it on a baking sheet. Sprinkle 3 tablespoons of olive oil. Dash a generous pinch of salt followed by pepper. It should form a nice coat. Bake for thirty minutes, so that the contents become golden brown and soft. Take out and keep aside. Lower the oven temperature to 375 degrees Fahrenheit/190 degrees Celsius.

5. For Tofu Filling: Drain the tofu. In a food processor, place the drained tofu, salt, pepper, and hummus. Blend and set aside.
6. Mix in a bowl the veggies you have baked in the oven along with the tofu mixture. Stir and form a coating. Add the crust to this and form a smooth layer.
7. Bake this quiche in the oven which is now preheated at 375 degrees Fahrenheit/190 degrees Celsius. When d2, the quiche has the golden brown top layer, which also is firm. It takes around thirty to forty minutes for this. If the crust turns dark brown, tent the edges with foil.
8. Let the quiche get cooled for a few minutes. Serve with green onions or fresh herbs.

Chickpea Nuggets

Ingredients:

- 1 can Garbanzo beans

- 1 cup bread crumbs

- Frying oil

- Seasonings: roughly 2 tsp of each

- Garlic powder

- Onion powder

- Salt

- Pepper

- Oregano

- Basil Seas2d salt

Directions:

1. Add all Ingredients: to food processor and mix to consistency similar to dough. (Can be mashed and mixed by hand)
2. Mold nuggets and fry in hot oil for about 30-45. seconds on each side. Eat with your favorite dipping sauce!

Bean Tacos

Ingredients:

- 1 can pinto beans

- Choice of fresh toppings (use this opportunity to pile as many fresh vegetables as possible into the tortilla!)

- Above: lettuce, red onion, tomato, yellow bell pepper, cilantro.

- Tortillas

Seasonings:

- 2 tbsp cumin

- 2 tbsp chilli powder

- 2 tbsp salt

- 2 tsp cayenne

Directions:

1. In a sauce pan add can of beans and seasonings.
2. Saute for about 3 minutes. Use potato masher to smash beans to a "refried" bean consistency.
3. Add beans to tortilla and pile on fresh toppings!

Chickpea Scramble Breakfast Basin

Ingredients:

For chickpea scramble:

- A drizzle olive oil

- ½ tsp salt

- 1 can (15 oz.) Chickpeas

- ½ tsp turmeric

- 2 garlic cloves, minced

- ½ tsp pepper

- ¼ white onion, diced

For breakfast basin:

- Handful parsley, minced

- 1 avocado, wedged

- Handful cilantro, minced

- Greens, combined

Directions:

For chickpea scramble:

1. Scoop out the chickpeas and a little bit of its water into a bowl. Slightly mash the chickpeas using a fork, intentionally omitting some. Stir in turmeric, pepper and salt until adequately combined.
2. Sauté onions in olive oil until soft, then add garlic and cook for 1 minute. Stir in the chickpeas and sauté for 5 minutes.

For breakfast basin and serving:

3. Get 2 breakfast basins. Layer the bottom of the basins with the combined greens. Top with chickpea scramble, parsley, and cilantro.
4. Enjoy with avocado wedges.

Vegan Smoothie

Ingredients:

- 3 tbsp or 50g firm silken tofu
- 200ml (1/2 tall glass) unsweetened soya milk
- 100ml (1/4 tall glass) cherry
- 2 tbsp porridge oat
- 1 cherry soya yoghurt
- 75g (1 empty yoghurt pot) frozen cherry
- Juice

Directions:

1. Measure every 2 of those elements just or use a tall glass together with your empty yoghurt kettle for speed, they don't have to be exact.
2. Set them in a blender and blitz until smooth. Pour 1 tall glass or 3 short tumblers.

Quinoa, Oats, Hazelnut And Blueberry Salad

Ingredients:

- 1 cup oats, cut into pieces cups blueberries

- ½ cup dry millet

- ½ cup maple syrup

- 1-inch piece fresh ginger, peeled, cut

- 1 cup greek yoghurt

- ¼ tsp nutmeg

- 2 cups hazelnuts, roughl y chopped, toasted

- 2 large lemons, zested, juiced

- 1 cup golden quinoa, dry

- 3 tbsps olive oil, divided

Directions:

1. Combine quinoa, oatmeal and millet in a large bowl. Rinse, drain and reserve.
2. Add a tbsp of olive oil in a saucepan and place over medium-high heat.
3. Cook the rinsed beans for 3 minutes. Add 4½ cups of water and salt. Add the zest of 1 lemon and ginger.
4. When the mixture boils, cover the pot and cook over reduced heat for 20 minutes. Remove from heat.
5. Let stand for 5 minutes. Uncover and sponge with a fork. Discard the ginger and place the grains on a large baking sheet.
6. Allow cooling for 30 minutes.
7. Transfer the beans to a large bowl and mix with the remaining lemon zest.
8. Combine the juice of both lemons with the remaining olive oil in a separate bowl.

9. Add yoghurt, maple syrup and nutmeg. Pour the mixture into the beans and stir. Mix cranberries and hazelnuts.
10. Refrigerate overnight, then serve.

Tofu Club Sandwich

Ingredients:

- 1 avocado, peeled, pitted, sliced
- 2 teaspoons dried rosemary
- Tahiti, as required
- Salt to taste
- Pepper to taste
- Few fresh basil leaves
- 4 cloves garlic, minced
- 8 -12 slices bread of your choice, toasted
- 2 packages tofu, cut into slices of 4-5 mm
- Few lettuce leaves

- 1 cup onion or shallots, sliced

- 2 tomatoes, sliced

- Cooking spray

Directions:

1. Place a large nonstick pan over medium heat. Spray with cooking spray.
2. Add garlic, onions and rosemary. Sauté until onions are translucent.
3. Add tofu slices and cook until golden brown. Flip sides and cook the other side too.
4. Apply thin on the bread slices.
5. Place lettuce, mustard, avocado, tomato and tofu in the order menti2d on half the bread slices.
6. Top with the remaining bread slices.
7. Cut each club sandwich into 2 triangles and serve.

Italian–Style Spaghetti Squash With Tempe

Ingredients:

- 2 cups packed baby spinach

- 4 tablespoons tamari

- 4 cloves garlic, finely chopped

- 2 tablespoons canola oil

- 4 cups broccoli, cut into small florets

- 24 ounces tempe, cut into small cubes

- ½ cup miring
  2 spaghetti squashes (2.5 pounds each), halved lengthwise, deseeded

- 2 jars (25 ounces each) pasta sauce

Directions:

1. Place the squash with its cut side facing down in a large baking dish. Add 1-cup water.
2. Bake in a preheated oven at 375°F for 30-45 minutes or until the squash is tender.
3. Meanwhile, add Tempe, tamari, garlic and miring into a bowl.
4. Toss well and set aside for 30 minutes. Drain.
5. Place a large skillet over medium high heat.
6. Add Tempe and cook until golden brown.
7. Stir once in a while. Remove on to a plate and keep warm.
8. 6 minutes until crisp as well as tender.
9. Add spinach and stir. Remove from heat.
10. When the squash is d2, remove from the oven and keep it with its cut side facing up. Let it cool.
11. Shred the squash with a pair of forks and place on a large serving platter.

12. Pour hot broccoli and sauce over it. Place Tempe on top and serve.

Mexican Zucchini Casserole

Ingredients:

- ½ teaspoon pepper powder

- 2 ½ tablespoons flaxseed meal

- 2 cups zucchini, shredded

- 2 jalapeño peppers, deseeded, finely chopped

- 1 small onion, chopped

- ¾ cup Bisquick baking mix

- 2 tablespoons fresh cilantro, chopped

- 2 tablespoons extra virgin olive oil

- 4 tablespoons nutritional yeast + extra for topping ½ teaspoon salt

- 2.5 ounces water

Directions:

1. To make egg substitute: Add flaxseed meal and water into a bowl and mix well.
2. Place in the refrigerator for 15-20 minutes.
3. Add zucchini, onions, cilantro and jalapeño into a bowl and mix well.
4. Add oil into egg substitute. Mix well and pour over the zucchini mixture. Mix until well combined.
5. Add Bisquick mix, salt, pepper, and nutritional yeast and stir again.
6. Transfer this mixture into a parchment paper lined or greased baking dish.
7. Sprinkle some nutritional yeast on top.
8. Bake in a preheated oven at 375° F for 45 minutes or until brown.

9. Slice and serve immediately.

Healthy Baked Eggplant Fries

Ingredients:

For fries:

- ¼ tsp. paprika

- ¼ tsp. ground cumin

- ¼ tsp. onion powder

- 2 tbsp. fresh lemon juice

- 2 tbsp. apple cider vinegar

- 2 cups whole-wheat seas2d breadcrumbs

- 1 eggplant, cut into strips

- ⅓ cup unsweetened plain soy yogurt

- 1 tbsp. dried parsley

- ¼ tsp. garlic powder

For dip:

- 1 cup unsweetened plain soy yogurt

- 1 tsp. dill

- 2 cloves garlic, minced

- 2 tbsp. lemon juice

- Fresh black pepper to taste

Directions:

1. Preheat oven to 450 degrees. Line 3 large baking sheets with a non-stick baking mat or parchment paper.
2. Cut the top and bottom off of your eggplant. Cut the eggplant in half lengthwise and then into quarters. Next, cut the eggplant quarters into slices roughly ¼ in. thick. Now cut the eggplant slices into strips roughly the size of French fries.

3. Combine yogurt, parsley, garlic powder, paprika, ground cumin, onion powder, lemon juice, and apple cider vinegar in a large bowl. Toss eggplant fries in soy yogurt mixture, coating evenly.
4. Place breadcrumbs on a plate and lightly coat eggplant fries with breadcrumbs. Spread out evenly on trays making sure they don't touch. Bake in preheated oven for 10-15 minutes or until golden brown and crispy. Turn halfway during baking to brown evenly. Serve immediately with lemon dill dipping sauce.
5. For dip
6. Combine all Ingredients: in a medium-sized bowl. Place in the refrigerator for a minimum of 1 hour to chill and allow flavors to combine.

Simple Tofu Scramble

Ingredients:

- 2 tbsp oil or margarine

- 1 tsp garlic powder

- 1 tsp onion powder

- 1 tbsp soy sauce

- 1/2 tsp turmeric (optional)

- 2 tbsp nutritional yeast

- 1/2 onion, diced

- 1/2 green bell pepper, diced

- 1 block tofu, drained and pressed

Directions:

1. Press your tofu to make it ready for cooking.
2. Then, slice the tofu into approximately 2 inch cubes.
3. Crumble it slightly to get the consistency you like for your scrambled tofu.
4. Next, heat the oil or margarine in a large skillet or frying pan and saute the chopped onion, pepper and crumbled tofu for 3-5 minutes, stirring frequently.
5. Next, add the garlic powder, onion powder and soy sauce and reduce the heat down to medium.
6. Cook the tofu for 5-7 minutes (stir frequently and add more oil if needed).
7. Finally, add the nutritional yeast and stir to combine well and make sure that your tofu is well coated.

Lentil Soup

Ingredients:

- 1 Tablespoon of olive oil
- 5 Diced scallions
- 3 Tablespoon of tomato paste
- ½ can of coconut milk
- ¼ Teaspoon of salt
- Brown rice to serve
- 1 Cup of red lentils
- 3 Cups of vegetable broth
- 1Small peeled and cubed sweet potato
- 1Diced carrot

- 1 Tablespoon of minced fresh ginger

- 2 Tablespoon of curry powder

Directions:

1. In a large saucepan, combine the lentils and the water; then let it boil for several minutes
2. Reduce the heat and add your sweet potato, the carrot; half the quantity of ginger and let simmer for 10 minutes
3. In a medium skillet, add the curry powder and toast it until it becomes fragrant. Remove the curry from the skillet once it is toasted and return your skillet to the stove then add the olive oil.
4. Add the ginger and half the quantity of the green onions to a skillet over a low heat and sauté for about 4 minutes
5. Add the tomato paste and then continue to cook it for about 2 minutes. Stir in the toasted curry powder and mix very well.

6. Add the paste of the tomato with the milk to the base of the lentil. Let the Ingredients: simmer for 20 minutes
7. Serve and enjoy a delicious soup with rice!

Carrot Soup With Pistachios

Ingredients:

- 1 Teaspoon of fresh minced ginger

- 2 Cups of cored and chopped Apples

- 3 Cups of Cauliflower florets

- 1 Cup of chopped onion

- 2 Teaspoons of Cumin powder

- 1 Teaspoon of Cinnamon

- ½ Cup of Pistachios

- 2 Tablespoon of Virgin Olive Oil

- 4 Medium, peeled and finely sliced carrots

- 1 Tablespoon of minced garlic

- ¼ Teaspoon of Paprika

- 1/8 Teaspoon of Allspice

- 1 Teaspoon of Salt

- 1 Pinch of Pepper

- 2 Cups of Vegetable broth

- 7 Tablespoon of water

- Cilantro for garnish

Directions:

1. Preheat the oven to about 400°F and toast the pistachios on a baking sheet for around 6 minutes
2. Transfer your toasted pistachios to a medium sauce pan and cover it with 1 cup of water; let the pistachios simmer for about 30 minutes by about 1 inch with water. Meanwhile, heat the oil into a large pan and add the garlic, the

carrots and the ginger; then cook for about 3 minutes.

3. Add the cauliflower, the chopped apples, the onion, the cumin powder, the cinnamon, the paprika, the allspice, the salt and a pinch of pepper; then stir and let it cook for about 5 minutes
4. Add your vegetable broth into the sauce pan and cover it; then let it simmer for around 20 minutes
5. Drain the pistachios and puree it with a blender with a little bit of water
6. Transfer the mixture of your tender vegetable mixture into bowls; then serve and enjoy with pistachios and cilantro

Vegan Tteokbokki

Ingredients:

- 2 tbsp. red chili powder
- Salt to taste
- 1 tbsp. olive oil
- Sesame seeds for garnishing (toasted)
- 2 cups vegan rice cakes(soaked for an hour)
- 3-4 green onions chopped
- 1-2 garlic clove grated
- 1 ½ tbsp. coconut amino

Directions:

1. Discard rice cake's water. (Soaked water)

2. Add rice cakes, salt, pepper, garlic and half of oil in a bowl, mix it well.
3. Heat remaining oil in a pan; saute onions and then add rice cakes, cook it for 5 min.
4. Then add coconut amino and cook it for additional 2-3 min.
5. Garnish it with sesame seeds and serve hot!

Vegan Creamy Cucumber

Ingredients:

- ¼ cup dill chopped

- ½ cup cashew nuts (soaked for an hour and drained)

- Salt and black pepper to taste

- 1 tbsp. lemon juice

- 1 tsp. vinegar

- 2 cucumber slices

- ¼ cup green olives sliced

- 2 tbsp. red onion chopped

- Water as needed

Directions:

1. Add all Ingredients: to the blender except cucumber, olives, onion and dill.
2. Blend until it smooth.
3. Now mix remaining Ingredients: with it.
4. Enjoy!

Banana Quinoa Bars

Ingredients:

- 2 and a half cup of mashed overripe bananas (around three large bananas)

- 2-third cup of quinoa (rinsed)

- 2 tsp. of vanilla extract

- A quarter cup of sunflower seeds

- Half a cup of walnuts (chopped)

- Half a cup of almonds (sliced)

- 3 cups of old-fashi2d rolled oats (gluten-free)

- Three-quarters cup of raisins

- A quarter tsp. of kosher salt

- 2 tsp. of ground cinnamon

- 3 tbsps. of maple syrup

Directions:

1. Preheat the oven. The temperature required is 350 degrees Fahrenheit/180 degrees Celsius.
2. Use a parchment paper to line the baking pan. The pan should be of 8X8 dimension.
3. In a food processor, make oats flour by blending for seven to ten minutes.
4. Mash the bananas in a big bowl.
5. To the bowl, add the other Ingredients: almonds, raisins, vanilla extract, sunflower seeds, walnuts, maple syrup, cinnamon, salt, floured oats, and quinoa.
6. Transfer the mixture to the pan, and spread as a smooth layer, and make it even.

7. Bake till the edges begin to turn mildly brown. This can take around 35 - 45 minutes. The bars should not turn brown.
8. They should be chewy and soft.
9. If they turn brown, it implies that they are burning.

Overnight Oats With Fruits

Ingredients:

- 2 tsp. of maple syrup

- 2 tbsp. of chia seeds

- A cup of frozen fruits of your choice (thaw them)

- A three-quarter cup of almond milk

- A half-cup of oats (rolled)

Directions:

1. Use a jar for keeping the thawed fruits and also use a spatula to mash them until pureed.
2. First, add the maple syrup and rolled oats.
3. Then, add the chia seeds, followed by the almond milk.

4. Use the lid to cover the mixture without stirring and keep it overnight in the fridge.
5. If you are meal prepping, you can keep it in the refrigerator for nearly 5 days.

Sheet Pan Veggies

Ingredients:

- Carrots

- Potatoes

- Onion

- Green beans (fresh)

- 3 tbsp Olive oil Seasonings:

- Salt

- Pepper

- Oregano

- Basil

Directions:

1. Preheat oven to 375 degrees F

2. Wash and chop veggies. Place them on sheet pan.
3. Drizzle veggies with olive oil. Sprinkle seasonings and toss veggies with your hands to evenly distribute.
4. Cover with foil and bake for 30 minutes.
5. Check and continue baking until potatoes and carrots are tender.

Vegan Chilli

Ingredients:

- Pinto beans (canned)

- Red kidney beans (canned)

- Corn

- Chopped red, green & yellow bell pepper (½ inch squares. About ½ cup of each color)

- 1 yellow onion (chopped)

- Green onion (garnish)

Directions:

1. In a pot over medium high heat, sauté onions, bell peppers, and corn in oil.
2. Once they become tender, add beans and seasonings.

3. Stir, cover and reduce heat. Simmer for about 15-20 minutes.
4. When beans have become soft, add green onion and preferred toppings.

Kiwi Fruit Smoothie

Ingredients:

- 1 pear, peeled, st2d and chopped
- 500ml lemon juice
- 1 banana, sliced
- 3 peeled kiwi berry

Directions:

1. Add each of the Ingredients: in a blender and blend until smooth then pour into 3 glasses.

Protein Breakfast Burrito

Ingredients:

For tofu:

- ¼ tsp salt
- 1 tsp nutritional yeast
- 3 garlic cloves
- 1 tsp oil
- ¼ cup parsley, minced
- ½ tsp chilli powder
- 1 tbsp hummus
- 1 package (12 oz.) Firm tofu
- ½ tsp cumin

For vegetables:

- ½ tsp chilli powder

- 1 pinch salt

- 5 fresh potatoes, sliced into pieces

- 1 tbsp water

- ½ tsp ground cumin

- 1 medium red bell pepper, sliced thin

- 2 cups kale, chopped

For assembling:

- 1 medium avocado, ripe, chopped

- 4 large tortillas

- Cilantro

- Hot sauce

Directions:

1. Preheat the oven to 400 f.
2. Squeeze out excess moisture from the tofu by wrapping it in a towel and placing a heavy object on top. Squash into thin pieces and set aside.
3. Place the potatoes and red pepper on a baking sheet lined with parchment paper, then sprinkle with water, cumin, chilli powder and salt.
4. Mix and bake for 22 minutes. At the 17-minute mark, add kale, mix and bake for an additional 5 minutes.
5. Preheat a skillet over medium heat. Add oil, garlic and tofu once the pan is hot, then sauté for 8 minutes, stirring frequently.
6. Meanwhile, mix hummus, yeast, chilli powder, cumin and salt in a bowl, then add 2 tbsps of water.

7. Add the parsley. Pour the mixture into the tofu and cook until lightly browned. Set aside.
8. Spread each tortilla and scoop out a large portion of the potato mixture, tofu mixture, avocado, cilantro and some hot sauce in the middle of each tortilla. Roll up and seal the seam, then serve immediately.

Vegan Cheesy Sc2s

Ingredients:

- 1 berry stalk

- 3 thyme sprigs, leaves picked

- 3 tbsps nutritional yeast

- 1/4 tsp mustard powder

- 250ml almond milk

- 300g self-rising flour, plus extra for dusting

- Vegan onion chutney

- 1/4 tsp smoked paprika

- 1/2 tsp baking powder

- 3 tbsps olive oil, plus extra

- 1 tsp white wine vinegar

Directions:

1. Heat the oven to 220oc and lightly grease the baking sheet.
2. Mix the vinegar with the almond milk and set aside.
3. Bring a pot of water to a boil, then add the cauliflower stem and then cook for 5 minutes until it is almost tender.
4. Drain well, let cool, and then chop finely.
5. Mix flour, baking powder, nutritional yeast, spices, thyme leaves and 1 tsp of salt in a large bowl.
6. Add the cauliflower, then add the oil and pour in 230 ml of this sour almond milk.
7. Working fast, bring the mixture with a wooden spoon; even when there is a dry mixture of the bowl, add more almond milk to create a smooth but not sticky dough.

8. Tilt the dough on a floured surface and touch to a depth of approximately 2.5 cm.
9. Trim the rounds with a 6 cm striated cutter and transfer them to the pan.
10. Gather all the cuts and cut more rounds.
11. Bake on the top shelf of the oven for 10-12 minutes until golden brown.
12. Drink hot with onion chutney.

Dilled Chickpea Burger With Spicy Yogurt Sauce

Ingredients:

- 7.5 ounces canned or cooked chickpeas, rinsed, drained ¼ cup shallots, minced

- 2 tablespoons fresh dill, minced

- 1-2 tablespoon dry bread crumbs

- 1 tablespoon tahini

- 1 tablespoon lemon juice

- Salt to taste

- Pepper powder to taste

- ¼ teaspoon ground cumin

- 2 tablespoons vegetable oil

- 3 pita pockets

For the sauce:

- ½ cup vegan yogurt

- 1 clove garlic, peeled, minced

- ¼ teaspoon curry powder

- ¼ teaspoon cayenne powder

- A large pinch salt

Directions:

1. Add half the chickpeas, tahini, lemon juice, salt, pepper, and cumin to the food processor bowl and process until smooth in texture.
2. Add remaining half chickpeas into a bowl and mash lightly. Add shallots, dill, lemon juice and bread crumbs.
3. Add the processed chickpea mixture into it. Mix well.

4. Divide the mixture into 3 equal portions and shape into patties.
5. Place a nonstick skillet over medium heat and add oil.
6. When theoil is heated, place the burgers and cook on both the sides until golden brown.
7. Stuff the burger in the pita pockets and serve with sauce.
8. To make the sauce: Add all the Ingredients: to a bowl and whisk thoroughly.

Lovely Vegan Flapjacks

Ingredients:

- ¾ cup (3 oz, 75 g) brown sugar

- 3 cups (9 oz, 225 g) medium oatmeal

- A pinch of salt

- ½ cup (4 oz, 110 g) non-dairy margarine

- 4 tbsp. light syrup (golden syrup)

Directions:

1. Oven: Pre-heat to 350F (180C)
2. Gently melt the margarine in a pan.
3. Remove from the heat, then add the other Ingredients: and mix thoroughly.
4. Pour the mixture into an oiled 8 x 12 in (20 x 30 cm) baking tin.
5. Smooth down the top with a fork.

6. Bake for 15 - 20 minutes.
7. Cut into pieces while still hot.
8. Remove from the tin when cold.

Mac & Cheese

Ingredients:

- 1/4 tsp. turmeric
- 1 1/2 cups "milk" (soy/rice milk)
- 1 cup shredded vegan cheese (cheddar/monterey jack blend)
- 1/2 tsp. mustard
- 1/4 tsp. black pepper
- 1 tsp. garlic powder
- 1 lb. cooked pasta shapes (large elbows, shells, etc.)
- 3 Tbsp. margarine
- 3 Tbsp. flour

- 1 1/2 tsp. salt

- 1 tsp. onion powder

Directions:

1. Cook pasta according to package Directions:.
2. In a small bowl, combine the flour, salt, pepper, garlic, onion and turmeric. Set aside.
3. Melt the margarine in a saucepot over medium/low heat.
4. Once melted, add the flour/spice blend and whisk in pot until combined.
5. Then add 1/2 cup of "milk" and whisk until smooth (no lumps!) After it thickens a bit, add another 1/2 cup of "milk" and whisk.
6. After a few minutes, add the remaining 1/2 cup of "milk" and whisk for several minutes until it thickens a bit.
7. Then add in the cheese and mustard and whisk regularly for about five minutes or so, until the cheese has melted into the sauce.

8. Pour sauce over freshly cooked noodles.

Quinoa Soup

Ingredients:

- ½ cup of corn

- 4 cups of vegetable broth

- ½ cup of water

- 1 can of drained chickpeas

- 1 can of diced tomatoes

- 1 tablespoons of tomato paste

- ¼ cup of dry quinoa

- 1 cup of chopped spinach

- ½ teaspoon of salt

- 1 pinch of pepper

- 2 teaspoons of olive oil
- 1 large diced onion
- 2 minced garlic cloves
- 2 diced large carrots
- 2 diced celery stalks
- 1 and ½ teaspoons of italian seasoning
- 1 and ½ cups of chopped green beans
- 1 pinch of salt

Directions:

1. Heat the oil in a large pan over a medium heat and add the onion; then cook for about 5 minutes
2. Add the garlic and sauté if for 1 minute
3. Add the carrots, the celery and the Italian seasoning; then cook for about 5 minutes

4. Add the thawed green beans, the thawed corn, the vegetable broth, the water, the chickpeas, the tomatoes, the tomato paste and the quinoa; then boil the Ingredients: on a low heat for 16 minutes
5. Remove the lid of the saucepan and lower the heat; then let simmer for about 20 minutes and stir from time to time
6. Add the spinach and stir very well; then adjust the seasoning and the salt with the ground black pepper
7. Serve and enjoy your soup!

Pumpkin Soup

Ingredients:

- 1 tablespoon of salt

- 2 teaspoon of pepper

- 3 tablespoons of coconut oil

- 2 lbs of raw pumpkin, raw

- 1 can of coconut milk

- 2 teaspoons of curry powder

Directions:

1. Turn on your stove to a medium heat coat a deep saucepan with 3 tbsp of coconut oil
2. Once the oil melts, add the curry powder and the pumpkin
3. Sprinkle the salt and the black pepper

4. Add the milk and the water until the pumpkin is covered and once it boils, reduce the heat and let the pumpkin cook until it becomes soft for about 20 minutes
5. Once your Ingredients: become tender, puree the Ingredients: with a blender and serve it with cilantro
6. Serve and enjoy a nutritious soup!

Vegan Spanakopita

Ingredients:

- ½ cashew cream
- 1-2 clove garlic grated
- ¼ cup ground walnuts
- ½ cup vegan butter (melted)
- Olive oil for brushing
- 1 pack vegan Phyllo pastry sheets
- 2 cups spinach chopped (frozen)
- 1 ½ cup vegan cream cheese

Directions:

1. Preheat oven to 375° F

2. Add all Ingredients: in a food processor except pastry and process it until well combined.
3. Brush pastry sheets and cut it into horizontal strips.
4. Place this stuffing at the corner of the strips and fold it in triangle shape.
5. Place it on lined baking sheet and brush it with oil.
6. Bake it for 15 min and enjoy!

Vegan Loaded Potato Bites

Ingredients:

- ½ tbsp. vegan cheddar cheese shredded
- Salt and black pepper to taste
- Vegan sour cream and chopped chives for garnishing
- 10-12 small potatoes (boiled)
- 4-5 vegan pepperoni chopped
- ½ tbsp. vegan butter

Directions:

1. Preheat oven to 400° F
2. Cut the potatoes into 3 halves and scoop out the inside.
3. Mix all the remaining Ingredients: with potatoes inside stuff.

4. Now fill potatoes with this stuffing and bake it for 10 min.
5. Garnish it with cream and chives.

www.ingramcontent.com/pod-product-compliance
Lightning Source LLC
Chambersburg PA
CBHW071456080526
44587CB00014B/2124